Calm in the Pain

Calm in the Pain

Table Of Contents

Foreword

Peace in pain," *A powerful guide for controlling your pain using natural method*" is an eBook that gives readers an insight on how to control pain by use of natural methods. Many people get themselves enslaved by pain or dependence on painkillers. This should never be so. There are a number of natural remedies that can be accessed free of charge all around our homes. These remedies are simple and good for a person's health. They also have minimal risks as supposed to pain killers.

In this eBook, we will look at what pain means. You will also get to understand what exactly happens in the body when you experience pain. This is very important. You have to understand what you are going through so as to know how to get through this. You also get some insight on how to determine the intensity of your pain.

In this eBook, you will also learn the different types of pain. When going through these different categories, try and determine what kind of pain you are having. If you aren't sure about your category, you can consult with your doctor. This is another important step in helping you understand your pain. It will also help you in identifying the right natural methods to use in controlling your specific pain.

This eBook will also give you some tips on what methods you can use to control your pain naturally. Based on your specific type of pain, there are a number of recommended remedies. As a precaution, ensure that you first talk to a doctor in order to find out which methods will be best suited for you. You are also advised to research more on each method that you select.

Finding the right method will help you minimize your pain and discomforts in a healthy manner and at a very low cost.

If you are wondering why it's important to try natural methods to control your pain as opposed to relying on pain medication, you will be able to find the answer to your question in this eBook. Some of the dangers of pain medication will be discussed in this book. At the end of it, you will realize that maybe rushing to the pharmacy every time you are in pain, is not really the best solution.

Controlling your pain using natural methods is very easy. Most people have tried out the methods discussed in the eBook and have managed to get very good results. However, there are some who have not been able to get their pain under control. The difference between these two groups of people is very simple. One group knows how to do it the right way while the other group is simply taking the wrong approach. This eBook takes a look at the do's and don'ts of pain management.

There are a number of common pains that many people undergo. In this eBook, we look at a few of this pains and how to control them. If you realize that your pain has not been discussed, you can carry out further research to establish which other the other natural methods discussed will actually work for you.

Peace in pain is very vital. If you let your pain stress you, this will only make your condition much worse.

Chapter 1:

An Overview of Pain

Synopsis

In this chapter, you will learn what pain means. You will also learn the impact of pain on your body.

- ➢ When a person is in pain, what exactly is going on in their bodies?

- ➢ Is pain just physical or can it also be psychological?

- ➢ Can you measure pain?

To know how to control your pain, you have to know what exactly happens to cause you this discomfort.

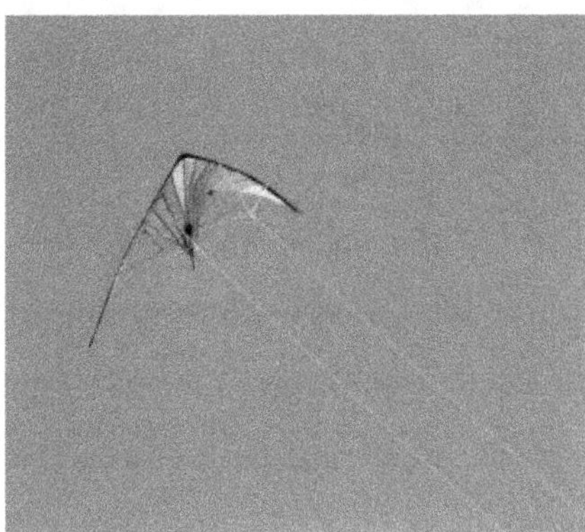

Basic Info

Definition of Pain

Pain can generally be defined as an unpleasant feeling. This is normally transmitted to the brain through the neurotic system. This feeling can be caused by an actual injury or even by a potential one. Once this is experienced in any part of the body, the signals are transmitted to the brain and interpreted as pain. This is what creates the physical awareness of the feeling and causes the person to react. This response can be physical or even emotional.

Pain may occur due to an injury such as a broken limb, a stabbing wound, a cut, a tear of the skin and a number of other injuries. The intensity of the pain may depend on the type of the injury and the extent. Pain may also occur as a result of an illnesses or medical condition. Examples of such pains include abdominal pain, chest pains, ovary pain headaches and a number of other pains. Pain may also be brought by psychological conditions such as depression. There are also times when someone may experience pain but the trigger is not identified.

When the pain signal is transmitted to the brain, this alerts a person to move their body from the cause of the pain. For instance, if someone steps on you, you will immediately experience a sharp pain. This will cause you to react and move away. If there was no serious injury, then the pain may easily go away immediately. However, if any tissue injuries occur, you may need to get some pain relievers in order to get rid of the pain.

It is always advisable to visit a doctor when you experience pain. This is much better than actually running to the pharmacists and getting off the counter pain. Pain may be a symptom for something more serious and that's why it should never be ignored. Once you have consulted with a doctor, then you can enquire about the natural methods that you can use to control the pain. Remember, it's not wise to start with the natural methods without first seeing the doctor.

A doctor will advise you on the best methods to use to control your pain.

Pain can affect a person's ability to take part in the daily activities. For instance, it may affect the ability of person to move around especially with limb pains. In serious cases, pain can seriously affect a person ability to live normally. There are things like excitement that may actually worsen the individual's pain. Depending on the type and intensity of the pain, a person may not be able to live without pain medication.

Pain may be a symptom for something else.

Pain intensity

When you go to the hospital, doctors can use a scale to establish the intensity of pain. This is necessary to enable them to determine just how much pain you are currently feeling. This can help them determine the seriousness of your pain. It will also give them an indication of the amount and intensity of medication to be used. The pain scales can also help in indicating just how effective the medication is.

Pain scales can also be used for natural methods of controlling the pain. If you have been using natural methods, you can use the scales to determine whether the methods you have been using are working or not. You can get a scale to use at home or alternatively have a doctor use their scale for you.

Some of the scales that are normally used for this include, the number scale. This scale is from number zero to ten. Zero represents no pain, whereas the number ten represents intense pain. The intensity of the pain may fall to any of the other numbers between this.

There are also word scales whereby a patient normally uses words to describe their pain. They can describe it using adjectives such as severe, moderate or mild. There are also faces scales. These normally work best with kids. Different faces show different degrees of pain. A kid just has to pick out the face that best represents how they feel.

Chapter 2:

Synopsis

There are different types of pains. These categories will be discussed in detail in this chapter.

> ➢ What are the different types of pain and their symptoms?

Pain may be classified according to the intensity, duration and the part of the body affected. Other parameters that may be used in this classification include the system affected, symptoms and also the pattern taken by the occurrence of the pain.

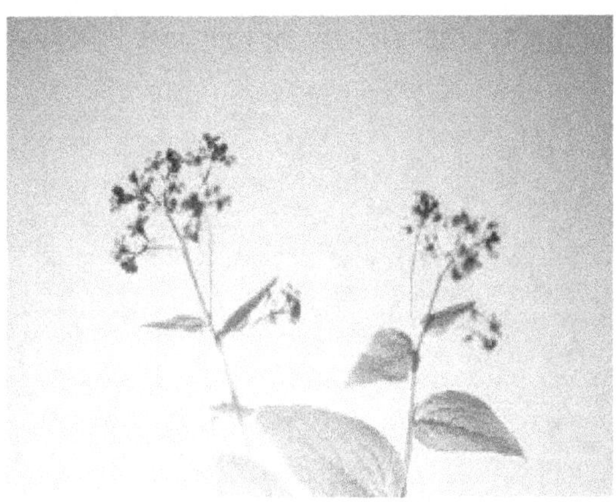

Chronic Pain

In a normal scenario, pain will only exist as long as the stimulus is present. Once removed, the pain normally goes away. However, in chronic pain, the pain may occur for long period of time. This may spread over a number of years although chronic pain is defined as any kind of pain that goes on for more than six months. This normally takes a toll on the patient physically and at times even emotionally.

Although chronic pain is considerably more serious, it occurs differently in different people. In some cases, it may be mild and may not really cause the patient any serious discomforts. In other cases, it may be very bad or excruciating .the pain may also be continuous or may occur in episodes. The intensity of the pain may also determine whether a person will be able to live normally or not .In worse case scenario, a patient will be immobilized and unable to perform any normal activities due to the pain.

Causes

Chronic pain normally occurs due to a number of causes. These include injury pains, chronic headaches, back aches, sinus pains, tendinitis, muscle pain, nerve pain, and carpal tunnel syndrome. There are also pains that may occur to particular parts of the body such as the chest, pelvic and others. There are also serious medical conditions that may cause chronic pain such cancer, ulcer, arthritis and others.

Physical Symptoms

Some of the symptoms likely to be experienced include:

- Pain that doesn't go away after a period of time. It may be severe or mild.

- Sharp, burning, shooting or electric pain.

- A feeling of discomfort that makes one feels some kind of tightness, soreness, stiffness or aching.

Associated Symptoms

There are some symptoms that normally occur as a result of the pain. These include disability, insomnia, fatigue, low immunity, mood changes. All these symptoms will go away once the cause of the pain is established and subsequently eradicated.

Consequences

Chronic pain if not properly controlled can have some serious consequences on a patient's life. It may take a toll on a person's finances if medication is relied on. It may also have psychological implications on a person.

One of the main results of this pain is depression. Dependence on pain medication has the risk of addiction. Statistics show that the addiction to painkillers is on the rise especially among young people. The pain may also inhibit a person. They may not be willing to take part in any activities that may possibly cause them pain.

Chronic pain may also inhibit the cognitive ability of an individual. It impacts on their memory making them more forgetful. It also affects a person's ability to concentrate on a task. A person may also appear to be distracted. In some cases, it may also affect a person's speech abilities.

Remember, if you have chronic pain, you have to first consult a doctor. Don't try out natural remedies until a doctor has correctly identifies the stimulus for the pain.

Once this is done, you can then seek counsel on the best methods to use to control the pain naturally. You don't have to suffer for the rest of your life due to the pain. There are things that you may be able to do from your home to minimize the suffering in just a couple of months.

Acute Pain

Acute pain normally starts very sharply but it doesn't last for so long as in the case of chronic pain. Acute pain normally signifies a problem in the body. It may also be brought about by different circumstances. For instance, labour pain. These pains are very sharp and may cause one a lot of discomfort.

However, they may last only a couple of hours. Sometimes a cute pain may simply be mild and only lasting a few minutes. In most cases, acute pain can be treated in just a couple of months. Once the stimulus is identified and eradicated, a person will be ok again.

Under the acute and chronic pains, there are two further subdivisions for pain. These are Nociceptive and neuropathic pain.

Treatment for Acute pain

Most people tend to turn to pain medication to treat acute pain. This is because this pain can be sharp causing one such discomfort that they may want to get rid of very fast.

However, there are a number of other natural methods that can be used to control this pain. Some of the most popular methods include, massage, physical therapy, breathing exercises, psychotherapy, music therapy and also distraction therapy. It is always advisable to consult the doctor before getting started on any natural alternatives.

Nociceptive pain

If a bone or muscle is injured, a person is likely to experience nociceptive pain. Nociceptor basically refers to pain sensors. These are what transmit signals to the brain alerting about the pain.

A person experiencing this kind of pain may be able to exactly point out where it is coming from. It normally feels like it's only in one area and may not affect the whole body. Normally this pain goes away after a short while. However, in cases like arthritis, it may take a while to go away.

Neuropathic pain

This type of pain normally occurs around the nervous system often as a result of undergoing an operation or getting injured. Many people describe this kind of pain as burning, pin pricking, electric shock or very sharp pain. Touching the area around the nerves normally escalates the pain. This pain may last for months or even years.

Psychogenic pain

Emotions and other mental factors can actually cause pain. They can also make the pain continue for period of times. One of the most common examples of such pains is headaches. However, stomachaches may also be psychogenic. If this pain becomes chronic, it may easily cause depression in a patient.

Phantom pain

This type of pain is normally experienced by amputees. It revolves around the body part that was lost. The duration and intensity of the pain normally differs ion different amputees. In some of them, it lasts only for a short period after the amputation .In others it may go on for a period of months or even years. The pain also varies in intensity. In some it's really severe while in others it remains like a mild irritation.

People who have lost a limb are likely to experience pain referred to as, phantom.

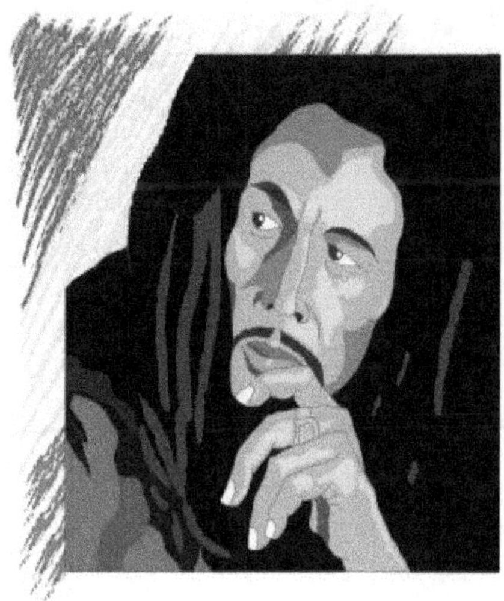

Chapter 3:

Synopsis

You don't have to run to your doctor every time and get painkillers. In this chapter, we look at some of the natural methods that you can use to control your pain.

> ➤ How can you control your pain without medication?

Using medication for prolonged period of times can be very harmful to your body. If you experience any pain, you can first consult your doctor and ask about alternative natural methods that you can use.

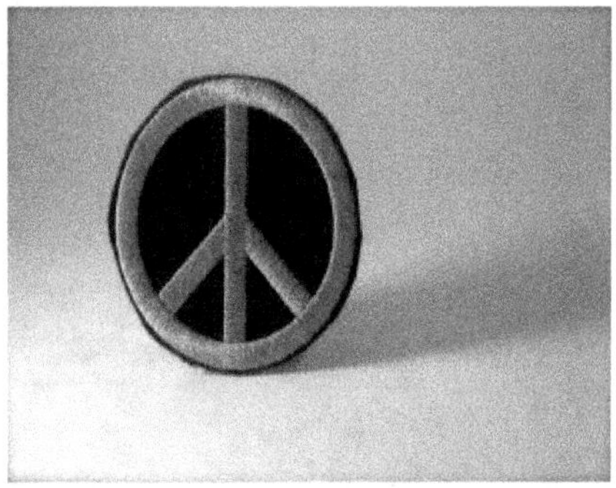

Natural Ways

Acupressure

Acupressure is one of the most common natural methods for pain relief. This simply works by applying pressure on some specific parts of the body depending on the pain that one experiences. Remember, the spot that you will rub isn't the spot where the pain is. Different spots work for different parts of the body.

You have to identify the right spot for the acupressure to work. If you don't, you will notice that your pain will not work even after repeated efforts.

Techniques to use

There are two main techniques for administering acupressure. The first one is by applying pressure to specific spots. The second technique actually works in the opposite. You have to reduce pressure on the specific spot.

You have to use something blunt to apply the pressure. Some people use their fingers but this may not be very effective. In addition, you will have to apply the pressure for prolonged periods of time so as to get the desired effects. However, if you have to use your fingers, ensure that you use the tips or the nails. Thickness may affect the procedure. Ensure that whatever you decide to use to apply the pressure is less than 4mm in thickness. The pressure has to be applied for at least a minute. However, even after just a minute, the effects will already be felt. Don't press too hard as you may hurt yourself. At the same, if you do it so lightly, it will not work.

The second technique involves making anticlockwise motions with your figure on the pressure point. You can repeat these motions for about two minutes. Like in the first technique, you will start to feel the difference in just a matter of seconds. However, it is not advisable to do this for long periods of time.

Applying pressure at the right point can help relieve pain. You can do this with the tip of your finger.

For some people, acupuncture also works. The acupuncturist will place the needles on spots depending on the location of the pain. These placements help in the release of a chemical called endorphin. This is the chemical that gives a person, the feeling of peace and euphoria. It can easily shift the focus point from the pain. However, like in the case of acupressure, you have to first check with your doctor before attempting to use this method.

Hot packs or cold packs

This strategy is commonly used to relieve headaches. The hot and cold packs aren't just used for headaches. They also work very well for muscles aches. They can help get rid of the pain in just a matter of minutes. You can also find some of the gel packs that are normally reusable. Some of these are normally present in most of the first aid kits. You can also find specific packs that are designed for specific injuries.'

In place of the packs, people also use cherry pits. These are used the same way the packs are. You just have to place them on the area that is affected in order to get some relief. Cherry pits are popularly used to treat pains in areas such as the back, the neck, joints and even headaches. They can also be used to bring relief to areas affected by arthritis. Research shows that you can also use the cherry pits on your acupressure points to give you some relief from pain.

Body massage

A full body massage may help you get rid of any pains in your body. You can also get massage for specific parts of your body that may be in pain. For instance, in case of back aches, you may decide to get a back massage to relieve this. Massaging the area helps in regulating the circulation of blood in the area and therefore getting rid of the pain.

You can have a friend massage you. However, you should also consider hiring a professional to do it. This is because they are normally trained for the job. They know exactly what to do to relieve the pain that you may be feeling. Massages are also good for relieving the stress that may occur due to the pain. This normally happens especially when someone has chronic pain. Massages are also very good when it comes to relieving pain around the joints. This is because they relax the muscles and therefore ease the pressure around the joint.

A massage can help you in getting rid of pain.

Meditation

This is another good technique in helping get rid of pain. It helps the mind focus on other things apart from the pain.

Herbal remedies

There are so any different types of herbs that are well suited for pain relief. In fact most of the painkillers that people buy are actually made from herbal extracts.

One of the most popular herbs for pain relief is the willow bark. This is actually the key ingredient in aspirins. This herb has an ingredient known as salicin. Once ingested into the body, these changes to another component called salicylic acid. This is the key component that works in relieving pain. This herb can work for both chronic and acute pains.

Turmeric is also great for controlling pain. This herb is especially preferred for controlling arthritis pain. You can add turmeric powder to your food. Menthol offers a good natural pain reliever. This is very effective especially for muscle aches. You can find extracts from this herb to rub around the painful area. This will give you relief in just a matter of minutes.

Getting rid of stress

Freeing your mind from stress can also help you in controlling your pain. In most cases, stress actually makes pain much worse. There are so many different ways that you can relieve your stress. These include, getting new hobbies, exercising, listing to nice slow music, talking to someone, meditation, yoga, reading a nice book and getting rid of the stressor. For instance, if you are in a relationship that is stressing you, getting rid of this stressor may be quite helpful for you. If the stressor is your work, you can try and talk to your management team to see what can be done. Whatever you decide to do, you have to ensure that you get rid of your stress. This is what will help you control your pain.

Deep breathing exercises are also very helpful especially in helping one relax. This can be very good in the relief of pain. Breathing exercises are also a great choice for chronic pains such as mid low back pains.

You should also try and ensure that the area that you live in is clear and free of anything that may stress you. Avoid living around clutters either at work or even at home. Always ensure that you stay in rooms that have plenty of air. This may mean opening up your windows for periods of time. Clean fresh oxygen is also good for the relief of pain.

Exercise

There are some types of pains that can be controlled by exercises. With the right type of exercises, the pain may also be reduced considerably and even in some cases completely eradicated. This especially works for muscles pains and for limb pains as a result of an injury. However, these exercises have to be keep very light so as not do more harm. For instance, with a painful hand, simple hand motions can provide good exercises. On the other hand, trying to lift weights or use a punching bag will only make things worse and can cause further injuries

Light exercises are also good for people who are suffering from arthritis. At first, the exercises may bring about some pain and discomfort. This may especially happen if the limb had been left to rest for sometime without any exercises. However, after a few times, the pain may start fading away. Patients are however encouraged not to strain themselves. If the exercises prove to be too painful, one should stop them or consult with a doctor.

Carrying outs just simple exercises can greatly help in the control of pains especially around the joints and also the muscles.

Hypnosis

Did you know that hypnosis is effective in the reduction of pain? Well, according to studies, it is. More than 70% of the people who use this technique for pain release can attest to its effectiveness. Hypnosis works for people who are experiencing chronic pains and also for the acute pains.

Meditation is also very effective in controlling pain naturally. When one relaxes their mind, they will learn how to shift focus from the pain. If someone is suffering from acute or chronic pain whether severe or mild, meditation can help them relax and completely ignore the pain. Concentrating on the pain often makes the situation worse. Meditation normally requires some amount of discipline. One has to practise every single day. You have to set aside a time and place for this exercise. Find an area free from distractions or any other type of interruptions. One technique of meditating is focusing the mind on the breathing patterns. You can do this even for half an hour during which you shouldn't think of anything else but the breathing. You can also mediate on positive affirmations. An example of such an affirmation is "I am stronger and able to get through anything". Try and get good affirmations that don't even mention the pain at all. You have to ensure that your mind stays away from that.

Protective Gear

There are a number of protective gears and other things that can help minimize pain especially in limbs. These are things that can be used to minimize mobility until the limb heals. Such protective gear includes splints and braces. These are especially suited for joint pains. This can reduce pain around the joins and avoid straining them to the point of causing further injury. In case of broken limbs, it's also good to keep them elevated so as to encourage the circulation of blood into the limbs.

Berries

There are actually berries that can be used to help in the reduction of pain. One such berry is from the chaste tree. This is an excellent remedy for acute pains such as the relief from muscle cramps resulting from menstruation periods. If you normally have painful periods, try eating these berries for your next three periods. Studies show that this normally relieves the pain by more than 50%.Apart from the cramps; the berries will also help in the relief of other PMS-symptoms such as mood swings, headaches, back aches and breast tenderness.

Saunas and Hot Tubs

Many people think that saunas and hot tubs are mainly meant for just having a good time. However, what most people don't know is that they can also be very good in offering relief from any kind of muscle pains. The heat from the saunas and tubs normally facilities the circulation of blood in the body. This helps in soothing the areas affected.

Fruits and Vegetables

You should ensure that you eat a balanced diet rich in fruits and vegetables. You especially require Omega 3 for pain relief. You should also drink plenty of water. When it comes to foods rich in Omega 3, fresh water fishes such as salmon and sardines is highly recommended.

On the other hand, it is strongly recommended that you stay away from eating foods that contain a lot of fats, sugars or even salts. These may result in inflammation which can make the pain worse. Other foods to avoid include meat, refined food, pork and junk food.

Fresh water fishes rich in Omega 3 fats also provide relief from pain.

Fish oil is highly recommended for controlling back pains, joint pains and also arthritis.

Music

Music is actually great for pain relief. Research shows that listening to good soothing music reduces pain by almost 20%.The music is also great for taking one's mind away from the pain. This helps in relaxation and pain relief. Music is great for relieving acute pain such as labour pains or any pains resulting from surgeries.

Music is a great natural method for controlling pains. In addition, it helps in getting rid of some of the psychological symptoms that come with chronic pains such as depression, anxiety and disability. It helps the mind to relax and not focus on the pain.

Yoga

Yoga has a number of benefits to the body. One of the main benefits is controlling and minimizing pain such as arthritis and migraines. Yoga is also a powerful tool for meditations. It helps in the relaxation of the mind. This is another reason why it's very helpful for people with chronic pains especially.

Yoga is also a great natural method for controlling mid low back pain. It helps in exercising the body through stretches. It also helps in making the body more flexible and stronger. Yoga is cost effective and has such a wide range of benefits in the overall health of the body and the mind.

Yoga is good in helping in the control of pain. It relaxes the mind and helps in the stretching of muscles.

Life style Changes

Patients can make a few life changes to help in controlling pain. Things like alcohol and coffee aren't good for pain management. You can do away with these or at least cut down. Smoking can also be really bad when it comes to the management of pain. These three normally stress the body tissues making the pain worse. You also have to eat healthy and exercise so as to keep your pain in check. Being overweight can also make the pain worse.

Pets

Although there is no scientific proof to explain this, getting a pet can be good for controlling your pain. Pets helps ion improving the quality of life for an individual. These are actually good for people who may be suffering from orthopaedic pains.

Your pets may actually help in controlling your pain.

Capsaicin from chilli peppers

Capsaicin is an ingredient found in chilli peppers. If you round this on your skin around the painful area, it can offer you some relief from the pain. This ingredient can be found in form of cream. It's normally sold in pharmacies and drug stores. However, you don't need to get the cream if you can find the raw form of capsaicin.

Ensure that you don't use Capsaicin in open wounds or broken skin. You should also ensure that you don't rub your eyes with this ingredient. One of the main side effects of this treatment method is a burning sensation. However, this normally goes away after a short period of time.

A Bath

Did you know that a good warm bath can actually help in controlling pain? This is actually referred to as balneotherapy and is commonly recommended for chronic pains like on the mid low back. This method works well with mineral water and other Dead Sea salts. You can buy these in beauty shops or even drug stores. These baths are also provided in spas.

You have to ensure that you get clearance from your doctor before trying out balneotherapy. This method of controlling pain is actually not recommended for people who maybe having heart conditions.

A good bath in water that has the right type of minerals can help in controlling pain.

Chapter 4:

Synopsis

The dangers of using pain medication.

There are so many people who are completely dependent on painkillers. In this chapter, we look at some of the dangers that may arise due to this overdependence.

> What are the effects of relying on pain killers?

> What are the dangers of using pain medication for long periods of time?

It's never advisable to keep running to the chemist for pain medication every time you feel any kind of pain. You may actually be doing more harm than good to your body.

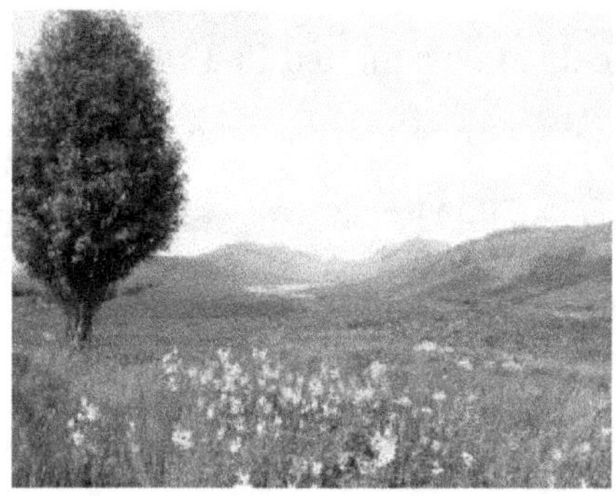

What Can Happen

Addiction

One of the most serious effects of using painkillers for a long period of time is addiction. A person may depend on the medication so much that it becomes hard to live normally without the medication. In addition, the prolonged use may cause one to become tolerant to the medication. This may push them to increase their dosages so as to get any pain relief.

Addiction normally occurs over a period of time. One of the ways to know that you are getting addicted to the medication is when you start abusing it. This abuse may occur inform of over or under dosages. In addition, you may find yourself using the painkillers even if not in pain.

Addiction to pain killers is just as serious as being addicted to heroin. It can ruin a person's life. It gets them alienated from friends and relatives. It also prevents them from concentrating on other things such as their careers. Addiction may also lead to death in case of over dosage. This problem normally leads patients to be admitted to a rehab centre so as to get over their addiction. Sometimes one may become an addicted knowingly but at other times, some people don't even realize that they are addicts until it's too late.

Kicking this habit is very hard especially because of the withdrawal symptoms. Some of these symptoms chills, nausea and vomiting, headaches, muscles pains and many other symptoms. These normally vary according to the individual and other factors such as the degree of addiction.

The risk of addiction doesn't just fall to the patients but also to the people living with them. According to statistics most addicts are normally in their teen years. Further studies show that these teens normally start experimenting with painkillers when they are available in the house. This is normally due to the ease of availability. For this reason, parents are advised to keep their pain medication away from the kids. They should also throw away any pain medication that is currently not being used.

It is very easy to get addicted to pain killers.

Cardiac Arrest

Research shows that many people who use pain medications for long periods of time are likely to have a cardiac arrest. Taking a lot of these medications normally interferes with the normal breathing processes. This affects how the heart pumps blood to other body parts and may lead to problems of blood circulation in the body. Massive cardiac arrest may easily cause the death of a person.

You can get a heart attack if you use pain killers for a long period of time.

Drug Interactions

There are some people who tend to use more than just one painkiller at a time without knowing the dangers of this habit. This interaction is normally dangerous and has been known to cause death in a number of situations. Mixing the painkillers with other drugs or supplements may also be fatal. Mixing the medication with alcohol or even coffee may also be very dangerous.

Abuse of Painkillers

One of the most abused pain medications is Oxycontin. This is an active ingredient that is normally found in most painkillers. One of the ways to abuse the medication is by use of the wrong methods of ingestion. Although the medicine is supposed to be ingested orally abusers ingest it in powder form through sniffing or by mixing it into a soluble form and ingesting through injection.

Over Dosage

There are so many reported cases of deaths through overdose of painkillers. In some cases, this is normally done intentionally whereas in other cases, it may be done accidentally. A person who intends to commit suicide through painkillers will just simply take as much as they can. This is easy to do especially when painkillers are readily available and if the person is not in their right frame of mind. Many people who suffer from chronic pain and depression are at risk due to this. The person who is taking the medication is not the only one likely to commit suicide. Sometimes, having painkillers around friends or relatives who are depressed may actually tempt them to take their own lives. This is one of the reasons why people are advised to keep their medicine locked away.

Overdosing accidentally is also a major risk. This normally happens when one starts abusing the painkillers. If you feel the need to increase your dosages just so as to get some relief, then you run the risk of overdosing. Also, if you feel like your normal dosage doesn't work fast enough, and then you are likely to overdose. Over dosage is also likely to happen to people who have developed tolerance to the medication due to the prolonged use of pain medication. Some of the symptoms that come from over dosage of pain medication include, nausea, vomiting, chills, general body weaknesses .In the worse case scenarios, the patient may have liver failure, cardiac arrest and die.

Side Effects

Many painkillers have a number of side effects that normally vary from one individual to another. Some of the common side effects include nausea, vomiting, itching, dry mouth and drowsiness. Other serious side effects include gastrointestinal pains. These can be mild or very serious resulting to ulcers or internal bleeding of the stomach walls.

Other side effects include, frequent urination or pain when passing urine. Painkillers may also cause urinary tract infections especially in women. A patient may also feel constipated.

Financial Strain

Trying to control chronic pain by sue of painkiller can be very expensive. This is especially the case when one tries to acquire the medication without a prescription especially in the case of addicts. Trying to hide the habit may also be very effective. It is also very expensive to keep buying over the counter medication even when dealing with acute pains. Instead of spending so much money purchasing medicine, it is much better to try out the cost effective natural methods which aren't likely to harm one's body in the long run.

Chapter 5:

An Overview of the Do's and Don'ts of Controlling Pain Using Natural Methods

Synopsis

In this chapter we look at some of the things that you should do when you want to control your pain through natural methods. At the same time, we will also look at some of the things that you should never do.

> ➢ What should I do when I am in pain?

Natural methods of controlling pain will only work for you if you do them right. If you don't do the right thing, you will not help yourself. In addition, you may actually make the pain worse.

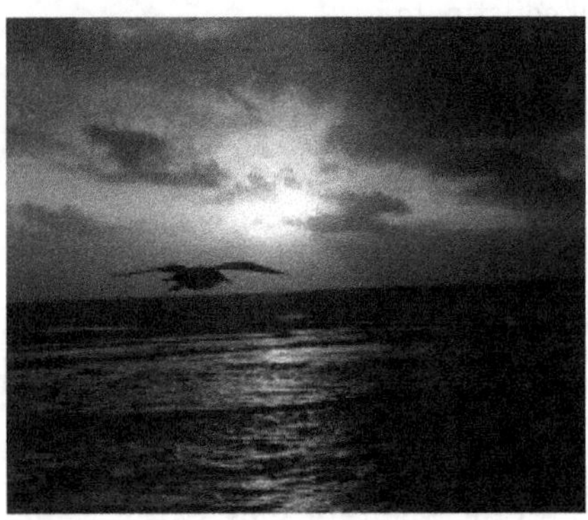

What To Do

The Do's

When you are in pain, you do have to see the doctor. The natural methods will come after this. This is especially the case with severe pain whether acute or chronic. For instance, if you get injured, consult with a medical profession first. Don't just stay at home and start of the natural treatments.

The doctor will be able to assess the degree of your illness and pain. This will help them in advising you on the right kind of treatment methods to use. At this point, you can ask the doctor about the right natural methods to use for your pain.

Some of the natural methods may not be suitable for you. This is the same way; some medications may not be suitable for individuals due to certain reasons. For instance, you may find that some herbs may not agree with your body. There are also some types of exercises that may not work well for you due to the nature of your pain. All this information will be availed to you once you go and see your doctor.

Consistency

Like in any kind of treatment method, you have to learn how to be consistent with the kind of natural method that you decide to use for pain. It will not be likely to work if do it just once. You may get instant results for a while and then the pain comes back again.

For instance, if you decide to make changes on your lifestyle by cutting down on coffee, alcohol and also smoking, you can't just do this for a short period of time then once the pain subsidizes, you go back to your usual returns. This will not be helpful; to you. The same applies to exercises and other returns. For example, if you want to use yoga, you have to do this severally. You can't do it once a month or once in every two weeks. You have to make this a part of your routine.

You will not be able to control your pain unless you commit to your treatment method. Result is not likely to come instant but they will be felt once you keep repeating the control methods.

Research

Once you know that you have a specific kind of pain, do some research about it. There is so much credible information that can give you tips on how to control your pain. Read and consult widely and ensure that you learn as much as you can. In your research, find out the list of natural methods that you can use. Once you identify these, you then need to research on each specific method. In some cases, you will find other details such as side effects and allergic reaction. You will also find useful information and how to best use the natural methods.

One of the places where you can kind this information is on the internet. For instance, if you have back pains, just conduct an online search on natural remedies for beck pains. You will find a lot of articles and other published materials on these. Compare the information that you get from different sources and identify the best control methods.

You can also find very valuable information by reading books. For instance, this eBook gives you an insight on some of the methods that you can use to control your pain. It's now up to you to dig deeper. Carefully research on each of these methods to determine which ones will best suit you.

Medical professionals also offer very valuable research. Talk to your doctor or anyone else who practices medicine. Remember, to be accurate in the information that you give them. Describe your pain and don't forget to fully disclose your medical history. If you have any illnesses or allergies, you have to tell the doctor so as to enable them to give you the right advice.

Reading more about the pain and the methods to control is will be very helpful to you.

The Don'ts

Don't rush to the pharmacist and buy pain medication immediately you feel any kind of pain. This is a solution that many people run to. However, pain medication may simply offer you quick temporary relief without really addressing the cause of the pain. In addition, these medications pose a wide number of dangers as discussed in this eBook.

It is better to go and see a doctor for a proper diagnosis rather than trying to self-medicate. In addition, your pain maybe signalling very serious medical conditions which could be fatal if they are not treated. For instance, cancer is one such condition that may first show up inform of pain.

You should never push yourself so hard or even ignore your body. If you try a method for controlling pain and you feel like the pain is getting worse you need to stop immediately. It could be that you are using the wrong pain relief methods. You may also be using methods that aren't suitable for your type of pain or medical condition. If you keep pushing yourself, you may do more damage to your body.

Pushing yourself by doing strenuous exercises can be harmful to your health.

You should never despair and give up if you feel that the method is not working fast enough. Like in any type of treatment, you have to give yourself time. In addition, you need to be realistic. You may find methods that will make the pain bearable without really eradicating it completely.

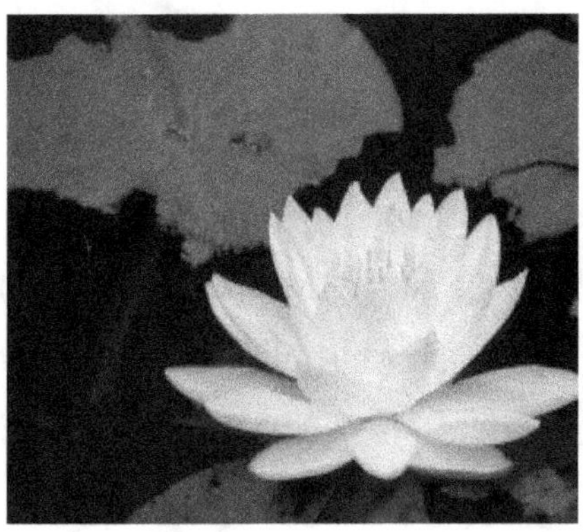

Chapter 6:

An Overview of the Recommended Remedies

Synopsis

In this chapter, we look at a number of natural methods for some of the most common body pains.

- ➤ What can I do to manage my pain?

- ➤ What natural methods can help me get through this?

For both acute and chronic pains, there are some specific natural remedies that can bring you some relief. These remedies may reduce the pain or even get rid of it completely.

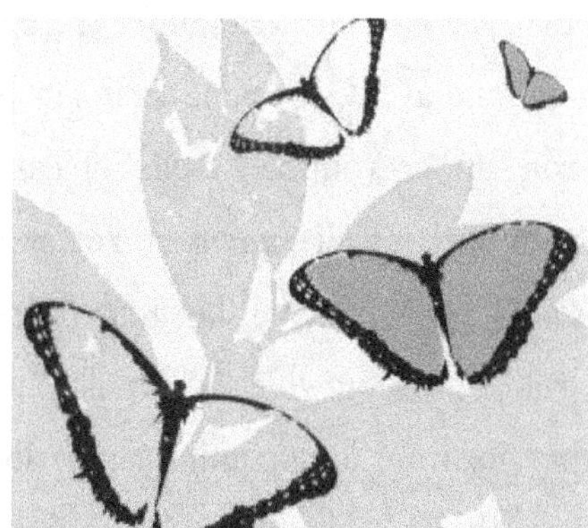

Some Help

Back pains

Many people suffer from acute or chronic back pains. This can be a result of sustained injuries or even medical conditions. There are also back pains that may be coming periodically. For instance, pregnant women and also women in the menstruation cycle may at times experience pain in the mid lower back for a period of time. Many people rely on pain killers to give them some relief. However, you don't have to do this. There are a number of natural methods that you can use to control your pain effectively.

Posture

You have to be very keen on your posture. If you have to sit down for long hours, ensure that you sit well to minimize the pains. You have to sit with your back straight and avoid slouching as much as possible. You also have to ensure that you support your back well. You can put a pillow on your seat to ensure that your back is well supported. You should also ensure that your knees and hips are level. When your knees are raised, your back will but put in an uncomfortable position which will make the pain worse. You should also avoid sitting down for long continuous periods. Try and take a break and stretch your body. This will offer you some relief.

Learn how to sit upright even when working on your computer. The wrong posture can make your back pains worse.

You sleeping posture will also contribute to aggravating or controlling your pain. If you want to sleep well, you have to sleep on your side. Try and bend your knees slightly and put a pillow between them. It is very important that you sleep on the right type of mattresses. This has to be firm enough so as to provide your back with adequate support. Using a bad mattress is one of the factors that contribute to back pains.

You should also walk in a good posture. Hunching your back will make the pains worse. Ensure that you keep your back straight and walk well. You should also maintain a good posture even when standing. Stand upright with your back straight. If possible avoid standing for long hours.

Lifting

When you want to lift anything heavy, try and bend on your knees keeping your back straight. You can easily do this by standing very close to the object that you want to lift. At all costs, avoid heavy lifting. You can easily do more damage to your back.

Back Pains in Pregnancy

There are a number of things that women can do to control their back pains especially during the initial stages of pregnancy. Some of the things that can help in alleviating this pain include, exercising by walking, pelvic rocking or doing min crunches. These are simple exercises that will not strain the body or make the woman fatigued.

Good posture is also mandatory in helping alleviate the back pains. This includes standing and sitting upright. No matter how comfortable slouching may seem, it is not advisable.

Simple exercises can greatly help in controlling back pain in pregnant women.

Yoga is also very helpful in alleviating back pains. It helps the woman stretch her muscles and avoid the pains. It is also recommended to get plenty of rest so as to avoid straining the body.

As a precaution, it is always advisable to consult a doctor about the best pain relief methods to use at different stages of the pregnancy. Some of the methods may not be well suited especially for the advanced stages.

Labour Pains

Most people think of labour pains as being an absolute nightmare of hours of never ending pain. However, you can actually control your pain through natural methods. This will help ease your discomfort through the whole delivery.

Water Birth

This is one of the natural methods of controlling labour pains. This is at times referred to as hydrotherapy. Women who deliver their babies through water births normally report that they experienced less painful contractions. However, it is wise to first consult with a doctor before selecting this birth option. There are women who may not be able to use this especially due to medical conditions or complications arising from the pregnancy.

Arthritis and Joints Pain

Arthritis and pain in the joints can be acute or chronic. There are few things that one can do in order to control the pain naturally instead of relying on pain killers.

One of the first things to do is to cut down on coffee, smoking and alcohol. This will prevent the occurrence of inflammation which normally worsens arthritis. People are also encouraged to also exercise the joints so as to reduce the pains. In most cases people try and keep the pints dormant in fear of feeling any pains. However, this is highly discouraged. Exercising the joints will make them more flexible and much stronger. This goes a long way in minimizing the pain.

You should also consider wearing braces or any other supportive gear such splints. This will prevent any unnecessary movements of the joints that may bring the pain. The supportive gear also helps in minimizing wear and tear. People who have arthritis are also encouraged to eat diets that are rich in alkaline. These include fresh fruits, leafy vegetables and foods that are rich in Omega 3.You should avoid taking junk foods and concentrate on eating healthy. This will greatly help in controlling the pain.

Sinus Pain

Many people suffer from chronic pains arising from sinusitis. However, there are some natural methods that can help such people in controlling their pains.

To control your pain, you have to learn how to eat and sleep well. This will help in making your immune system much stronger and therefore better prepared in fighting off sinus infections. Eating good food and getting plenty of rest also leaves your body well prepared in fighting off infections and therefore in minimizing pains. Avoid sugar foods as this will weaken your immune system.

Steaming is one of the methods that you can use to relieve the pain. There are many ways to do this right from home. You can use a hot shower and ensure that you close all doors to trap in the hot vapor. You can also pour hot water in a big bowl and then bend over it with a towel draped over your head to prevent the air from escaping. You can also use herbs to help in the steaming. Some of the recommended herbs to use include tree tea oil and lavender oil. Steaming helps in opening up nasal passages and easing the pain. It also helps in getting rid of the bacteria that normally worsens the sinusitis.

Acupressure also helps in controlling pain from sinusitis. The spot that you should put pressure on is between the thumb and the index finger on your left hand. You have to ensure that you find the area that will make a "V" shape. Use your right thumb to do this. For best results do this for about a minute or two.

You can also use salty water to clean your sinus. This is normally referred to as flushing. This normally helps in clearing the mucus buildup in the nose. You can also get rid of this mucus by eating spicy food. Try some hot salsa and you will find your sinus pain reducing considerably.

Flushing your sinuses with salty water can also help you in reducing the pain.

Chapter 7:

Synopsis

In this chapter, we look at some of things that can give you some peace of mind even as you work towards controlling your pain.

> ➢ What can I do to keep my pain from stressing me?

Peace of mind plays a key role in helping you control pain. No matter what method you select to use, with a stressful mind, you may not succeed.

Achieving Peace

Acceptance

Trying to deny the existence of the pain is very dangerous. You have to accept that you do have a problem that needs to be addressed. You can't ignore your pain forever. In addition, just because you refuse to acknowledge it, doesn't mean that it's not real. If the pain is permanent, accept it. However, acceptance doesn't translate to defeat. You just have to accept the pain in order to be able to get treatment or control methods for it.

In most cases, the denial occurs once a person has been diagnosed with a medical condition that may be considered as being serious. For instance, if you find out that the pain in your joints is caused by arthritis, the shock can lead to denial. However, once you accept that you have arthritis, and then you will be able to start looking for ways to control or treat your pain.

Distractions

You have to find ways to keep your mind off the pain. If you sit and wallow in misery, you will not be able to keep your pain in check. In addition, constantly thinking about the pain may actually make it much worse.

You may find distraction in finding new hobbies. If the pain normally limits your mobility, you can decide to find new hobbies that you can do without moving around such as reading or watching something. Whatever you do, don't let the pain keep you from living your life.

Watching TV or chatting with someone can help in getting your mind of the pain.

Socializing is also a good distraction. Talk to friends and family. Some people who have chronic pain tend to alienate themselves. This may be due to feelings of despair, anger or even bitterness. Other may be experiencing guilt due to the strain that their pain has on others. However, alienation is never a good decision.

Limit Your Research

There are people who tend to take their research a bit too far. It is good to read more about your pain. This may give you helpful tips on how to control it effectively. However, don't start obsessing on research. This may keep your mind focused on the pain at all times.

It may even do you more harm than good. On the other hand, some misleading information may even get you despaired. There is a lot of negative energy everywhere. Some people may be trying to spread this negativity to others. For instance, you may find information online that tells you the worst case scenarios for your pain. You may also get misleading information telling you that you can never be in control of your pain. Limit your research and avoid such materials. If you have any causes for concern then consult your doctor.

Relaxation Exercises

There are a number of exercises that you can take to help you get some peace in mind. For instance, yoga is very helpful in meditation and relaxation. Normal exercises can also help one in attaining a good healthy mind. Meditation is also a very helpful tool in mind relaxation. It can also help an individual focus their mind on other things part from the pain that they may be experiencing.

Finding a way to relax your mind can help in giving you peace that is necessary in controlling pain.

Get some order in your life

Studies show that when you don't have peace in mind, you will also not have order in your life and vice versa. If at work, clear your desk and make it neat. If you have clutter this may also add you more stress. You should also do the same with your home. Make the environment around you convenient for relation. You should also identify a special area in your house that calms you. If you ever feel overwhelmed by stress or even just by your pain, being in this room will definitely help in giving you some relief.

Disorder can bring you stress. You need to remove all the clutter around you so as to have a clear mind.

Wrapping Up

Pain can get you down especially if you feel like there is nothing that you can do about it. Many people turn to pain killer addictions not by choice but because they feel like that they don't have any other choice.

However, you have to realize that there is also ways something that you can do. You don't have to be enslaved by your pain. You can actually find good natural remedies around your home that can help you control the pain.

Peace in mind

Getting stressed about your pain will not do you any good. You need to focus on other things. Find things that normally get you relaxed and then concentrate on them.

In addition, stressing over your pain actually makes it worse. Instead of sitting around feeling sorry for yourself, use this energy and find natural methods that you can use to fight the pain. You may even find techniques that may turn into hobbies. For instance, yoga is very interesting. Once you learn how to relax your mind, you will find yourself actually enjoying the routines.

Eat well

Eating a well balanced diet will go a long way in helping you control your pain. This will also make your body much stronger and increase your immunity against further stressors from infections. A good diet will also minimize your pain. There are foods that are well equipped in fighting pain.

Live your life

You don't have to stop living your life the way you want to just because of the pain. You have to be able to live your life normally. You can still have a family and a career even if you have chronic pains .However, to live your life to the fullest and be very wary of pain killer's addictions which have managed to ruin very many lives.

Research

There are so many natural methods that can work for you. You have to identify them. When you go to the doctor, don't just settle on pain killers. Talk to your doctor and ask about techniques such as acupressure and massages. You will find the best techniques to use.

Best wishes!

www.ingramcontent.com/pod-product-compliance
Lightning Source LLC
LaVergne TN
LVHW010258200726
843506LV00014B/3300